CHLOROPHYLL - GREEN IS HEALTHY

THE GREEN LIFEBLOOD - A DECISIVE HEALTH FACTOR AND ENERGY PROVIDER

PETER CARL SIMONS

Contents

Preface

Dear Readers,

One of the most underestimated vital substances[1] on the planet is chlorophyll. We often regularly take vitamins, mineral supplements and trace element supplements to support our health. Interesting to note, is that chlorophyll, an element crucial to our health, is hardly taken into consideration. At the same time, vegetables such as cabbage, common nettle, parsley or spinach - all rich in chlorophyll, land less and less frequently on our kitchen tables, and when they do, are prepared in a way that depletes these wonderful sources of its rich and valuable nutrients.

The experience with nature shows that even predators (Carnivorans) cannot have a healthy existence without consuming plant products and substances. More and more, we encounter omnivores, like primates and humans. The steady decline of the consumption of natural plants, chlorophyll in particular, is a significant health risk as this substance is of extreme importance for healthy bodies. It strongly influences oxygen exchange in the cells, which is a basic function within our bodies and elementary for good health. That is why chlorophyll is also known as 'the green blood', for, as with blood, chlorophyll is necessary for survival.

In this book, I will show you the reasons why chlorophyll is crucial for your longevity and your health and how you can insure that your body gets enough of this wonderful vital substance.

I wish you a happy and healthy life!
Your,

Peter Carl Simons

[1]Wikipedia: »Nutrients act mainly as biocatalysts in cells and tissues in the presence of water, oxygen and carbon dioxide (the latter in plants) and are effective vital components. This includes, according to recent findings: enzymes, coenzymes, vitamins, hormones, exogenously-essential amino acids, exogenously-essential fatty acids, major and trace elements, fragrances and flavorings.«

ONE

CHLOROPHYLL – THE DISCOVERY

Joseph Priestley[1], an English scientist, discovered photosynthesis[2] in 1771. His research was continued by other scientists. Jan Ingenhousz recognized the importance light plays in photosynthesis.

Jean Senebier discovered the importance of CO_2 in photosynthesis, Théodore de Saussure the role of water and Julius Robert Mayer discovered plants convert sunlight into chemical energy during photosynthesis, which is the basis for plant life.

When researchers discovered chlorophyll[3] had a similar structure to hemoglobins in blood[4], speculations arose, that chlorophyll may be of similar importance to human health. These speculations have since been corroborated. During his research, German chemistry nobel prize winner Hans Fischer[5] (1881-1945) achieved groundbreaking results in this area.

Early on, there were attempts to implement his research. During the 1940s, people with artificial anuses were given chlorophyll to reduce odors. Chlorophyll was also given to people with trimethylaminurie_[6] Despite the fact that not all cases achieved the desired results (i.e. not in 100% of the cases), the positive outcomes outweighed the lesser positive results. You may often have heard about the household remedy to swallow a chlorophyll tablet [or eat a sprig of parsley] after consuming garlic or similar foods. That basically derives from the afore-mentioned approach.

[1]Wikipedia: »Joseph Priestley (born March 24, 1733 in Birstall in Leeds, England; † 6 February 1804 in Northumberland County (Pennsylvania), United States) was an Anglo-American theologian of Unitarianism, philosopher, chemist and physicist. Priestley described for the first time the representation and action of oxygen. He discovered display options for numerous other gases such as nitrogen dioxide, carbon monoxide, hydrogen chloride, ammonia, hydrogen sulfide, sulfur dioxide, silicon tetrafluoride "

[2]Wikipedia: »Photosynthesis or photosynthesis (old Greek φῶς Phos> light <and σύνθεσις Synthesis> composition <) is the production of energy-rich materials from lower-energy substances using light energy. It is operated by plants, algae and some bacteria. In this biochemical process, light energy is converted into chemical energy by the light-absorbing dyes using chlorophyll or bacteriochlorophyll. This is then, among other things, used for the construction of high-energy organic compounds - used in low-energy, inorganic substances, mainly in carbon dioxide CO_2 (carbon dioxide assimilation) and water H_2O - very often carbohydrates. Since the energy rich organic materials are components of the organism, their synthesis is referred to as assimilation.«

»In the 18th century it was known that animals could not survive in sealed glass containers. Priestley found that plants were able to survive well in sealed glass containers. Priestley examined together with the Dutchman Jan Ingenhousz (from 1779), the formation of gas, depending on the lighting conditions (photosynthesis). He also tried experiments with the resulting gas, which he called dephlogisticated air (oxygen). A mouse survived in this closed gas atmosphere and a burning candle did not extinguished. Priestley himself inhaled the gas, experiencing improvement in the chest cavity. Priestley recognized the toxic nature of exhalation many living things on earth, and the benefits of plants: The damage to the atmosphere constantly inflicted by exhalation by such a large number of living things ... and by the decay of plant and animal materials are , at least partially, counterbalanced by plant growth.«

[3]Wikipedia: »First descriptions of> color fabric <[sic], the (> alcohol <) can be extracted by ethanol and is decomposed under the influence of light, can be found at Heinrich Friedrich Link in his book> principles of the anatomy and physiology of plants', Göttingen 1807. Likewise, one finds ambiguous evidence that Joseph Proust had had the green dye described as> fécule <. Pierre Joseph Pelletier and Joseph Bienaimé Caventou had extracted the substance again, naming it chlorophyll. Initial studies on the chemical structure of chlorophyll had derived from Richard Willstätter (1913). The chemist Hans Fischer used Willstätter's research in the 1930s, and by 1940 he was able to clarify the structure of the molecule. Fischer's research results in 1960 were confirmed by Robert B. Woodward's chlorophyll synthesis.«

[4]The chemical structure differs from the central atom in chlorophyll magnesium and hemoglobin iron only.

[5]Wikipedia: »Hans Fischer (born July 27, 1881 in Höchst am Main; † March 31, 1945 in Munich) was a German chemist and physician. For his work> on the structural composition of the blood and vegetable dyes and for the synthesis of hemin <Fischer was awarded the 1930 Nobel Prize in Chemistry. (...) Fischer continued the work begun by Richard Willstätter's [sic] research on chlorophyll. 1940 he was able to clarify the structure of the molecule. His research results were confirmed in 1960 by Robert B. Woodward's chlorophyll synthesis.«

[6]Wikipedia: »Patients with Trimethylaminuria or the so-called 'fishy odor' syndrome smell like old fish. They secrete abnormal amounts of body fluids such as sweat or urine and trimethylamine.«

TWO

CHLOROPHYLL – OUR GREEN BLOOD BROTHER

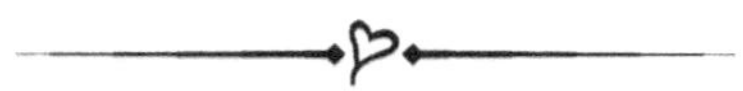

As previously stated,chlorophyll and hemoglobin share a similar chemical structure. Despite the complexity, the only difference between the two is the central atom. Hemoglobin contains the iron atom (Fe) which enables respiration and the transportation of oxygen throughout our system, while chlorophyll has magnesium (Mg) as the main atom. This difference allows plants to convert carbon dioxide (CO_2), exhaled by humans and animals, into oxygen (O_2) again.

Chlorophyll has the ability to absorb sunlight and transform it in a way that the human body can utilize it. The ensuing energy can in turn be used by humans. The simplest way to do so: chew on chlorophyll-rich plants which find its way into the body through saliva, an optimal way for the body to absorb it.

THREE

APPLICATIONS FOR CHLOROPHYLL

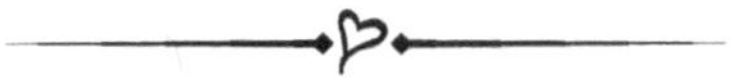

Many researchers, doctors and healers from around the world have added to the afore-mentioned rostrum of the countless positive effects chlorophyll has for human health.[1]

Anti-Aging

Chlorophyll has the ability to bind free radicals, assigning it the ability to prevent some degenerative diseases and premature aging. Research results indicate a life-extending effect.

Cancer Prevention

Clinical studies have shown that chlorophyll stymies the growth of cancer cells. In addition to that, it reduces carcinogenic effects found in packaged food and our environment.

Detoxifying Effects

Chlorophyll detoxifies the body, aiding the body to expel toxic substances, unhealthy foods as well as fighting off infections.

Hematopoiesis or the Formation of Blood

Chlorophyll stimulates the formation and cleaning of blood. The oxygen content is regulated which contributes to general well-being.

Body Odors

Chlorophyll neutralizes many body odors. Positive results are achieved in the battle against bad breath, foot odor, sweating in the genital region and armpit area, as well as odors caused by constipation.

Bowel Cleanse

Chlorophyll has positive effects on our bowel. It cleans the digestive tract and promotes bowel peristaltic_[2]. People who regularly consume chlorophyll rarely suffer from constipation. Residue of fecalith, cadaverine, odoriferous, rotting and acidic wastes are considerably reduced.

Parodontosis

Parodontosis is a challenge many face despite regular dental hygiene measures. The industry offers an array of toothpastes and mouthwashes to combat bad breath, yet many of us realize - despite these preventive measures - we are prone to pockets, up to one centimeter in size. And in these pockets, anaerobe bacteria flourish (in particular aggregatibacter actinomycetemcomitans_)[3], largely responsible for bad breath.

Research shows, that sulcus fluid excretes into these gum pockets. It is a by-product from the bowels and is transported through the bloodstream. Well-known scientists see a connection to the processes of anaerobic digestion and rotting waste, determining that the infections can be cleared through the ingestion of chlorophyll.

In turn, the body can begin to deal with the gum pockets and they begin to close up. Gargling regularly with dissolvable chlorophyll in water reduces gum bleeding in most cases.

De-acidification

It is common knowledge, that people in our cultural circles suffer over-acidification or acidosis. We consume more and more food that result in acidosis. Even fruit and vegetables don't contain the same PH values as they did prior to industrialized farming. Air pollution has led to acid rain, which in turn has a negative effect on the entire farming industry. This in combination with the fact that we are ever more sedentary, we sweat less (less excretion of excess acidity through sweat) resulting in extremely high PH factors.

Chlorophyll has a positive effect on our PH household. To achieve optimal results, experts recommend taking it throughout the day.

The Body's Water Balance

A balanced water household is important for our health and well-being. As we age, the body loses its water reserves i.e. it becomes more difficult to retain the necessary fluids in our bodies. The resulting effects: our blood gets thicker, the cells decrease in size and cell membranes shrink. Brain volume also decreases as well as the elasticity of body tissues decrease.

The daily call to drink more often falls on deaf ears, especially amongst people over 50. Why? The more you drink, the more you have to run to the bathroom and sadly, the trip to the bathroom increases as our water household storage capacity decreases. The latest research suggests that here too, chlorophyll exerts a positive influence on the body's ability to store water. Simultaneously, experts have witnessed an improvement of blood flow, which, in turn reduces the risk of a stroke.

Being Overweight

Paracelsus [4] knew: »You are what you eat.« Recent scientific studies draw the following conclusions: the wrong bowel bacteria are a direct causality of overweight. Naturally, this is not the only cause of overweight. Studies have shown, however, that people who consume more than the average amount of meat have more rotting bacteria in their intestines. Overconsumption of carbohydrates in form of bread, for example, has negative effects, resulting in an overpopulation of fungi bacteria.

Fungal infestation often leads to uncontrollable cravings, resulting in eating too many sweets. New studies have proven this, leading to the assumption that what we eat (the state of our bowel flora) also influences how we think. It is not without reason we speak of the bowel brain, since after the brain, the bowel contains the most nerve cells. Animal testing has proven that certain bowel bacteria changes behavior.

Regular bowel cleanses integrating the use of chlorophyll gives the body a chance to rid itself of rotting bacteria and fungi, allowing healthy bowel flora to thrive and is conducive to a healthier body. This is often the reason why some people lose weight after bowel cleanses.

More Areas of Usage and Side Effects

Several studies-, research- and experience- reports list many more beneficial effects that chlorophyll has. Some examples where the use of chlorophyll reduces healing time, lessens damaging effects: open wounds heal, sinus infections, orthodontic procedures and tooth extractions, depression and depressed moods, laryngitis, ulcers, bowel infections, blood sugar levels reduction, as well as fighting against iron-, magnesium and other deficiencies.

One must be aware that the use of chlorophyll, along with some of the other plants listed in this book can have adverse effects. Allergic reactions are possible,(especially when applied topically), food incompatibilities and related respiratory and digestive problems. Other side effects are conceivable.

For these reasons, it is always a good idea to consult your doctor before using any chlorophyll products. Your doctor should be clear, that reports extolling the virtues of chlorophyll are not cure-alls or promises to cure certain diseases or illnesses. Each body is different and reacts differently to different substances.

[1]Caution: we do not recommend self-medication. The use of vital substances and alternative remedies should always be done after a consultation with your physician.

[2]Wikipedia: »In contrast to the more uniform peristalsis of the small intestine, the large intestine contents are driven by periodic mass movements. They occur about once to three times per day in the colon and propel the intestinal contents forward to the rectum.«

[3]Wikipedia (en): »Aggregatibacter actinomycetemcomitans (previously Actinobacillus actinomycetemcomitans) is a Gram-negative, facultative nonmotile, rod-shaped oral commensal often found in association with localized aggressive periodontitis, a severe infection of the periodontium, although it is also associated with non-oral infections. Its role in periodontitis was first discovered by Danish-born periodontist Jørgen Slots, a professor of dentistry and microbiology at the University of Southern California School of Dentistry.«

»Bacterium actinomycetem comitans‹ was described by Klinger (1912) as coccobacillary bacteria isolated together with Actinomyces from actinomycotic lesions of man. It was reclassified as Actinobacillus actinomycetemcomitans by Topley & Wilson (1929) and as Haemophilus actinomycetemcomitans by Potts et al. (1985). The species has attracted attention because of its association with localized aggressive periodontitis.«

[4]Wikipedia: »Philippus Theophrastus Aureolus Bombastus von Hohenheim, baptized as Theophrastus Bombastus of Hohenheim (* probably in 1493 [1] in Egg, Canton Schwyz; † September 24, 1541 in Salzburg), called Paracelsus, was a physician, alchemist, astrologer, mystic, lay theologian and philosopher. The knowledge and work of Paracelsus is considered extremely comprehensive. Its

healing successes were legendary, but also earned him bitter hostility by established physicians and pharmacists, exacerbated by the often scathing criticism Paracelsus hurled at the prevailing doctrine of humoral pathology after Galen and the bookish wisdom medical scholars had at that time. Paracelsus left numerous German-language books and records of medical, astrological, philosophical and theological content, most of which were not published until after his death.«

FOUR

CHLOROPHYLL – NATURE'S PROVIDER

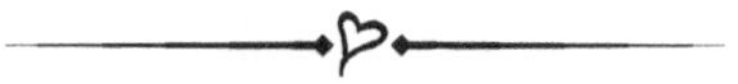

Chlorophyll can be found in almost every plant with varying degrees of concentration. Wikipedia provides a list of popular plants common to Central Europe and are listed in descending order according to their chlorophyll content.

	Chlorophyll *a*	Chlorophyll *b*
green cabbage	189 mg	41 mg
common nettle	185 mg	173 mg
parsley	157 mg	55 mg
spinach	95 mg	20 mg
broccoli	26 mg	6 mg
green beans	12 mg	4 mg
green Peas	10 mg	2 mg
cucumber	6 mg	2 mg
kiwis	1,7 mg	0,4 mg
white Cabbage	0,3–1 mg	0,1–0,2 mg

The chart shows that the common nettle contains the highest amounts of chlorophyll a and b, about 10 times higher than that of broccoli. Of plants grown in Europe, green cabbage belongs to those with the highest chlorophyll content.

Naturally, it makes sense to try and get your source of chlorophyll from freshly-harvested plants. However, products that are veritable chlorophyll bombs are available during the winter months too. The upcoming products offer a welcome supplement for a well-rounded, healthy diet during the winter months when fresh produce is not so readily available.

AFA – Blue Green Algae

The AFA or blue-green algae are also known as Aphanizomenon flos-aquae. Wikipedia describes its content:

The AFA-Bacteria 20 (of 25 known in the human body) contains amino acids, including the eight essential amino acids. In addition, the cyanobacterium has enzymes, vitamins, minerals and trace elements, known as co-enzymes and are part of enzymes. AFA contains beta carotene (provitamin A), most of the B vitamins and vitamin E. Furthermore, the AFA-bacteria has, relative to the total substance, more essential fatty acids than seeds, nuts and seaweed. For example, they contain almost as much gamma-linolenic acid (GLA) as breastmilk.

The scientific name of AFA is Aphanizomenon flos-aquae. The available products derive almost exclusively from the Upper Klamath Lake in Oregon (USA). The lake sits at 1262 meters above sea level. According to current research, Upper Klamath Lake is the largest remnant of a much larger pluvial lake that existed during the Pleistocene period, which began about 2.5 million BC. Through the surrounding volcanic rock formations and many other influences, the water contains a unique mineral composition. The AFA-algae has concentrates of twenty amino acids, vitamins, enzymes and mineral elements.

Spirulina

Spirulina[1] - found on the shelves of various health food stores - is a micro algae, belonging to the blue algae, and is found in tropical or subtropical regions. Certain sources report, that this type of algae existed thousands of years ago in Latin America - the Aztecs harvested it as a nutrient source. The indigenous peoples living in the Chad Basin were also known to have had these algae cultures surrounding the lake.

More recent reports emphasize the plant's high content of vitamin B12. Other reports state the positive influence on cholesterol levels; conclusive findings have yet however, to be released.

Chlorella

Chlorella[2] was discovered relatively late. Its scientific traits as chlorella vulgaris were recorded 1889. Melvin Calvin used the chlorella vulgaris for his research of photosynthesis and was awarded the Nobel prize in 1961.

According to some reports, chlorella is preferred by patients prone to bloating and bowel problems as it contains a relatively small percentage of protein. Chlorella is also used in alternative medicine for amalgam removal and heavy metals detoxification. Germany has its own production site since 1999.

Wheatgrass

Wheatgrass is the most famous of chlorophyll providers not living in water. Despite the fact that wheatgrass has been around for centuries and has been used across many different cultures, for example by natural healers such as Hildegard von Bingen, only recently has this chlorophyll-rich source been experiencing a renaissance. Ann Wigmore's (1909-1994) extensive studies on the subject seem to have influenced this rediscovery of wheatgrass as she was a strong advocate of wheatgrass consumption.

One big advantage of consuming wheatgrass juice as a source of chlorophyll is the absolute freshness of the product. Chlorophyll can be consumed in its freshest state - alive - if you will (as opposed to algae tablets, for example) and is experienced as particularly gentle to the bowels and digestive tract. Furthermore, wheatgrass seems to have curative properties against fungi and rotting bacteria in the bowel and intestinal tracts. Regular consumption predicates these curative abilities of course.

As wheatgrass is made up of ⅔ chlorophyll, its properties in producing blood hemoglobins have positive effects providing oxygen and nutrients to the body's cells.

Barley Grass

Barley Grass[3]_, has been cultured for over 5000 in grain production. Various sources reveal that it was also consumed as a green plant. For example, one report states that the Babylonian ruler Nebuchadnezzar,(605 - 562 BC) who was banished for seven years, nourished himself solely from barley grass, to achieve health and cerebral clarity.

Dependent on the soil upon which it grows, barley grass indeed contains an impressive array of vitamins, minerals and amino acids. Natural medicine uses barley grass as a bio-catalyst for all metabolic processes. It is also used to battle high blood pressure. In China, barley grass and wheatgrass are important elements of annual fast and detoxes.

Alfalfa – Lucerne

Alfalfa or Lucerne (Lucerne is the name commonly used in the United Kingdom, South Africa, New Zealand and Australia) is a cultivated plant, existing for approximately 3000 years and was cultivated as feed for domestic animals.

In Central Europe, the name Alfalfa is used for marketing purposes which makes sense as nobody really wants to eat animal feed, do they? Unless it's known for its health benefits, of course.

In the Arabian world, Lucerne has been known and prized due to its vitalizing properties for centuries now. Lucerne contains many vital substances such as vitamins, minerals, trace elements and chlorophyll. Lucerne also regulates the PH household.

The consumer should be aware, however, that many no-name products from overseas do not attain to the same standards as Europe. Genetically modified alfalfa plants are allowed in the USA since 2005. Several other countries are allowing this development as well.

Ginkgo biloba

Ginkgo[4] is also known as a "living fossil", as it's the last survivor of its kind from ancient times. The tag 'living fossil' seems appropriate as this tree really does have fantastical vital forces. A ginkgo tree was circa one kilometer away from where the bomb had been dropped at Hiroshima. The tree survived and is alive and well to this day.

Traditional Chinese medicine use ginkgo seeds to help cure maladies such as asthma, TB (tuberculosis) and kidney ailments. Gingko leaves contain high dosages of chlorophyll and is used in geriatrics when concentration and memory lag. As we know already from previously-mentioned traits, chlorophyll acts as a blood thinner, allowing the blood to flow better into the tiniest capillaries..

In addition, ginkgo biloba has strong antioxidant powers - important for fighting off free radicals.

[1]Wikipedia: Spirulina is oxygen photosynthetic and contains only chlorophyll a, which is also present in plants. Since Spirulina belongs to the prokaryotes, which chlorophyll is not, however, as with the eukaryotic plant cell in organized structures, the chloroplasts, isolated, but is located in membranes, which are distributed over almost the whole cell. Spirulina is replaced by other pigments, which superimpose the chlorophyll-green, a green-bluish tint.«

[2]Source: www.chlorella-vulgaris.eu (4-2015): »Its composition makes chlorella a valuable food. In relation to the dry matter, it contains more than 50% proteins, it is rich in polyunsaturated fatty acids, minerals, fiber, vitamins and chlorophyll. The dry matter has up to 4% of the highest chlorophyll content of all foods. It produces no toxic metabolites or decomposition products. It also includes a wide variety of phytamines, including carotenoids, flavonoids, polyphenols, polysaccharides and glycoproteins. The content of these high quality natural ingredients is in line with the observation that the regular consumption of small amounts of chlorella (a few grams), out of sync body functions are normalized. These effects are not solely explained by the effects of nutrients, vitamins and minerals.«

[3]Wikipedia: »Due to the high nutrient content, it is also used as a dietary supplement. The leaves of young barley plants are freeze-dried. This powder is dissolved and ingested in cool water. The taste is somewhat reminiscent of diluted spinach.«

[4]Wikipedia: »Special extracts from the Ginkgo leaves are used. These desired active ingredients (ginkgolides, terpene lactones) are enriched, the undesirable substances depleted (especially ginkgolic). The Commission E denotes

the dry extract of ginkgo leaves with a drug-extract ratio of 35 1 to 67: 1; a content of 22 to 27% flavone glycosides and from 5 to 7% Terpenlactonen; and 5 ppm under ginkgolic. The definition of ginkgo dry extract (Ginkgo extractum siccum raffinatum et quantificatum) according to the European Pharmacopoeia is very similar. For the treatment of dementia, only such extracts are marketable in Germany. Most pharmacological studies were carried out with the extracts EGb 761 and LI 1370. In Ginkgo based supplements, such as from supermarkets or drugstores, the desired efficacy is unclear, since their quality is often questionable and scientific studies are lacking.«

FIVE

GREEN SMOOTHIES

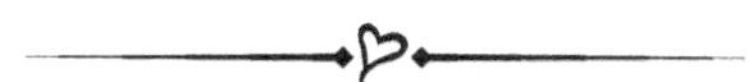

Green smoothies are becoming increasingly popular. This is a healthy trend because the ingredients are consumed immediately after production, and therefore oxidation is not a factor. This assumes, however, that the Green smoothies are home-made. Purchased drinks are - at best - a temporary solution.

Green smoothies are called "green", because the main components are high-content chlorophyll plants such as spinach, kale, broccoli, parsley,wheat or barley grass. The smoothies can be supplemented with fruit or other vegetables. Oranges, kiwis, apples, bananas, mangoes or pears are popular fruits used in smoothies. If you like, you can even add aloe vera gel.

Put all green plants etc. with water into a blender and mix. Green smoothies warrant a high-performance mixer with at least 25,000 revolutions. Only at a correspondingly high frequency are the individual plant cells 'opened', allowing for an 'unpacked' form of chlorophyll i.e. easily absorbed by the body. A conventional household blender is available for a fraction of the cost, but not suitable for producing/blending the kind of green Smoothies we're talking about.

SIX

WHAT YOU SHOULD WATCH OUT FOR

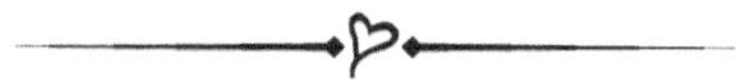

Browsing on the Internet, you'll find hundreds of chlorophyll products. If you add to that palette of products, further products containing spirulina, chlorella, wheat grass, barley grass or ginkgo, we easily reach the thousands.

It goes without saying that not all products are equal i.e. of the same quality. As I have stressed in my other advice books, I continuously warn against cheap no name brands. Many of these products don't contain the quality nor the quantity they state on the package. But what is much more egregious is the fact that these products often contain harmful additives that can, in some cases, induce allergic reactions.

If you buy or consume your chlorophyll from sources other than your own home-grown plants or from reliably organic sources, you should at least look for a reputable brand which identifies the ingredients detail. In addition, you should also consider the concentration of the desired vital substance, chlorophyll. In many cases, this explains the significant price differences and if you're in doubt, it's preferable to buy a more expensive product that contains decent amounts of chlorophyll rather than buying a cheaper product where you have to take triple the amount to meet your daily needs and achieve the desired results.

SEVEN

LITERATURE INDEX

- Arndt, U.: Spirulina, Chlorella, AFA-Algen: Lichtvolle Power-Nahrung für Körper und Geist, 2003, H. Nietsch
- Berner, H.-G.: An vollen Töpfen verhungern, 1997, Medi Verlagsgesellschaft
- Bertram, Dr. K.: Spirulina – Die Wunderalge – Anbau, Vorkommen und Zucht, sensationelle Studienergebnisse, Krankheiten vorbeugen und bekämpfen, o. J., Amazon Media
- Grillparzer, M.: Simple Detox: Das 7-Tage-Entgiftungsprogramm, 2013, Gräfe und Unzer, 5. Auflage
- Jester, F.: Arginin. Der natürliche Kraftstoff für Blut, Kreislauf und Gesundheit, 2010, Verlag Marina Jester
- Jester, F.: Chlorophyll – Das grüne Blut, Marina Jester Verlag, 2014
- Liebke, Dr. F.: Doktor Chlorella! Die Alge fürs Leben. Kompendium zur Mikroalge Chlorella, Remerc & Lheiw verlagskontor, 2007

- Loede, P: Schlank mit Weizengras: Die Gruene-Smoothie-Weizengras-Kur, Amazon Media, 2014
- Meyer, Marianne E.: Sonnenkraft mit dem blaugrünen Lichtträger Spirulina, 2002, Windpferd, 2. Auflage
- Mutter, Dr. J.: Grün essen!: Die Gesundheitsrevolution auf Ihrem Teller, 2013, VAK, 3. Auflage
- Opitz, Ch.: Befreite Ernährung, 2013, H. Nietsch, 5. Auflage
- Rahn-Huber, U.: Spirulina & Chlorella: Gesund und fit mit Mikroalgen, 2015, Riwei
- Simonson, B.: Gerstengrassaft: Verjüngungselixier und naturgesunder Power-Drink. Wildpferd, 15. Auflage, 2012
- Simonson, B.: Die Heilkraft der Afa-Alge – Vitalität für Körper und Geist, 2000, Goldmann
- Ulmer, G.A.: Gesundheitswunder Chlorophyll: Gespeicherte, gesundheitsspendende Sonnen- und Heilkraft, Ulmer, G A, 1997
- Wagner, W.: The Chlorophyll Supplement: Alternative Medicine for a Healthy Body, 2013, Health Collection
- Wolfe, D.: Superfoods – die Medizin der Zukunft: Wie wir die machtvollsten Heiler unter den Nahrungsmitteln optimal nutzen, Goldmann, 2015

Disclaimer

Introduction

By using this book, you accept this disclaimer in full.

No advice

The book contains information. The information is not advice and should not be treated as such.

No representations or warranties

To the maximum extent permitted by applicable law and subject to section below, we exclude all representations, warranties, undertakings and guarantees relating to the book.

Without prejudice to the generality of the foregoing paragraph, we do not represent, warrant, undertake or guarantee:

- that the information in the book is correct, accurate, complete or non-misleading.

- that the use of the guidance in the book will lead to any particular outcome or result.

Limitations and exclusions of liability

The limitations and exclusions of liability set out in this section and elsewhere in this disclaimer: are subject to section 6 below; and govern all liabilities arising under the disclaimer or in relation to the book, including liabilities arising in contract, in tort (including negligence) and for breach of statutory duty.

We will not be liable to you in respect of any losses arising out of any event or events beyond our reasonable control.

We will not be liable to you in respect of any business losses, including without limitation loss of or damage to profits, income, revenue, use, production, anticipated savings, business, contracts, commercial opportunities or goodwill.

We will not be liable to you in respect of any loss or corruption of any data, database or software.

We will not be liable to you in respect of any special, indirect or consequential loss or damage.

Exceptions

Nothing in this disclaimer shall: limit or exclude our liability for death or personal injury resulting from negligence; limit or exclude our liability for fraud or fraudulent misrepresentation; limit any of our liabilities in any way that is not permitted under applicable law; or exclude any of our liabilities that may not be excluded under applicable law.

Severability

If a section of this disclaimer is determined by any court or other competent authority to be unlawful and/ or unenforceable, the other sections of this disclaimer continue in effect.

If any unlawful and/or unenforceable section would be lawful or enforceable if part of it were deleted, that part will be deemed to be deleted, and the rest of the section will continue in effect.

Law and jurisdiction

This disclaimer will be governed by and construed in accordance with Swiss law, and any disputes relating to this disclaimer will be subject to the exclusive jurisdiction of the courts of Switzerland.